Natural Approaches
to
Healing Adrenal Fatigue

by Veronika Sophia Robinson

Natural Approaches
to
Healing Adrenal Fatigue

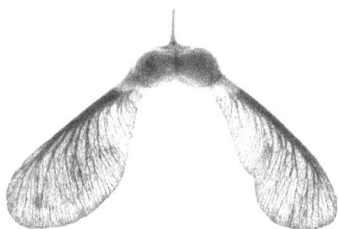

By Veronika Sophia Robinson

Natural Approaches to Healing Adrenal Fatigue
© Veronika Sophia Robinson
ISBN: 978-0-9560344-6-5

Published by Starflower Press
www.starflowerpress.com
July 2011

British Library Cataloguing in Publication Data.
A catalogue record for this book is available from the British
Library.

Also by the same author:
Fields of Lavender (poetry)
The Compassionate Years ~ history of the Royal New
Zealand Society for the Protection of Animals,
RNZSPCA
The Drinks Are On Me: everything your mother never told
you about breastfeeding (Starflower Press)
The Birthkeepers: reclaiming an ancient tradition (Star-
flower Press)
Life Without School: the quiet revolution (Starflower
Press), co-authored by Paul, Bethany and Eliza Robin-
son
Stretch Marks: selected articles from The Mother magazine
2002 – 2009, co-edited with Paul Robinson (Starflower
Press)
The Mystic Cookfire: the sacred art of creating food for
friends and family (Starflower Press)
The Nurtured Family (Starflower Press)
Howl at the Moon (contributing poet), Wild Women
Press
Peaceful Pregnancy CD, with Paul Robinson

For
Pam and Paul

The picture on the cover is of sycamore seeds, commonly known as 'angel wings'. These were chosen as symbolic of the homeopathic remedy used to treat adrenal exhaustion, and because this illness is a blessing in disguise; a wake-up call. It's as if the angels have come to visit and open our eyes to our current lifestyle.

Medical disclaimer:

The author is not a medical practitioner. The information provided within is based on her research and experience of healing adrenal fatigue naturally.

Neither the author nor the publisher is responsible for your experience.

~ Introduction ~

Unless you've had adrenal fatigue, it's very easy to dismiss it as 'all in the mind'. In fact, that's how most people who've experienced it are treated.

One Summer, I was driving along a motorway in the middle of day, hardly able to keep my eyes open. I hadn't had a late night, so what was wrong with me? I was so *exhausted*. Later that day, some friends came by, and I joined them in a cup of coffee. Ah, that's better! I felt great... but not for long. I'd made the usual mistake of thinking I was okay, but I'd just been momentarily propped up by an artificial stimulant. I spent the next month in bed, in a state of tiredness so achingly deep, that often I couldn't sleep.

My journey to discovering I had adrenal fatigue came about by accident (though, clearly, nothing is an accident), when I was looking up some information for the Italian translator of one of my books. During this research I noticed that a number of symptoms matched what I was experiencing. The jigsaw puzzle pieces started to fit together. Now that I knew what was causing 'Mrs Always Busy' to be flatlining, I could get to work and heal. The trouble was that most suggestions were alien to my lifestyle. I simply wasn't going to put adrenal tinctures from animals into my vegetarian body.

The next wake-up call came when we'd come back from a family camp for 40 families, which my husband and I organise. Paul is responsible for loading up the van with all the catering equipment, gas bottles, wholefood order, and so on. He's used to working, and spends as much time as I do on our magazine and proofreading books. After camp, he spent a few days in bed and was really run down. He had absolutely no energy. This fatigue went on and on and on, and it seemed hard to believe, but he too had developed adrenal fatigue symptoms. Two people in one family ~ a family with healthy eating habits. How could this be? We'd both been through the trauma of a court case, due to a right-of-way land disagreement, and as a result, later went through bankruptcy. We had month after month of incredible stress which was literally eating away at us.

This book is for those people who have adrenal fatigue and want to work with their body in a holistic way. I wish you a gentle and wholesome recovery. Go in peace. Be gentle with yourself.

~ What is adrenal fatigue? ~

Adrenal fatigue is most commonly recognised by the fact that rest or sleep does very little to relieve the symptoms, which are often seen as low blood pressure, irritability, depression, low blood sugar levels and a susceptibility to infections. We often learn to live with these symptoms, and don't tend to "hear" what's happening to our body until we can't stand up or function without coffee or other stimulants. This daily struggle to feel joyous about life is normal for those with adrenal fatigue. Negative emotions are inevitable when the body is in such a low state of energy.

There are various names for this state: adrenal exhaustion, fatigue, insufficiency; hypo function. This burnout is serious: *it 'rearranges' the body's natural energy systems.*

The adrenals are major glands. They're used by our body to respond to stress, commonly called 'fight or flight'. Stress produces the hormone adrenalin. They raise the blood pressure and blood sugar to ensure there is energy to respond to emergencies. This is all very good if we're in the jungle and need to run from a tiger, but when it's happening *every* day this leads to the hormones cortisone and cortisol being manufactured. The adrenals also produce aldosterone, which increases blood pressure and retains sodium. If we keep on triggering these hormones, eventually the adrenals become exhausted from overuse, and we can no longer handle stress of *any* description.

If you go to your doctor, s/he is quite unlikely to diagnose adrenal fatigue. Doctors generally don't have experience of recognising this illness, and only if enough tests are undertaken may they look for Addison's disease (the extreme end of adrenal exhaustion). When you've got adrenal fatigue, anything and everything triggers your 'fight or flight' response: the phone ringing, dog barking, electricity bill in the post.

Adrenal fatigue *is* curable, whether it's caused from a single trauma or has developed slowly. There are countless reasons for the cause of fatigue: stress, whether mental, physical, financial or spiritual; toxicity (chemical or emotional); nutritional mal-absorption. Stress requires our body to absorb more nutrients. However, most people reach for 'comfort foods' in the form of carbohydrates. These can create toxicity. Low protein in a diet can also impact on the ability to deal with stress. The adrenals require a diet rich in vitamins B, C, A, E, as well as the minerals zinc and manganese. Due to the poor quality of soil these days, many foods are deficient in minerals, such as selenium which is very helpful for alleviating painful joints and muscles.

We further deplete our foods by processing. Our 24/7 lifestyle means that many people don't take time to sit and eat a meal peacefully, perhaps dining by candlelight and gentle music. Instead, they're rushing from the door to the car or train, and scoffing down their food without much thought. This is wonderful for corporations like McDonald's, which literally feed off our time pressures, but our bodies are not designed to 'eat on the run'.

We live in a toxic world, where chemicals and heavy metals abound. These have a huge impact on the adrenal glands. On your journey to recovery you'll need to be conscious of every product used in your home, and put on your skin or in your body. Toxins can be found in toothpaste (fluoride), over-the-counter medications, dental work, household cleaning products, shampoos, etc. They're everywhere! But you can reduce and minimise how many are in your immediate environment.

Sadly, many children these days run the risk of adrenal fatigue, as they live a high-stress, fear-based and fast-paced lifestyle. Their bodies are bombarded by electromagnetic radiation: TV, computers, wi-fi, microwave ovens, mobile phones, sat nav, cordless phones, microwave towers, as well as unnatural noise pollution.

We survive on a diet of sugar, alcohol, coffee, chocolate and spicy foods to 'keep us going'. Other stimulants are: the news, thriller movies, rage, arguing, loud music, sexual stimulants.

People whose minds never switch off are just as susceptible to adrenal fatigue.

Worrying, being afraid or angry are not healthy responses to stress, and new habits need to be formed.

Children who've been conceived by parents with nutritionally-poor diets, are prone to burn out, even by three years of age. Symptoms include difficulty concentrating and depression.

There are many symptoms of adrenal fatigue. Copper levels rise, and zinc levels lower when the adrenals impact the immune system. Longer-term degeneration includes cancer, heart disease, Alzheimer's and Parkinson's. There are ways to detox and regain energy so that these diseases can be avoided.

Secondary to exhaustion are imbalance of the thyroid, PMT and hot flushes in menopause.

The reason people tend to become more emotional as a result of adrenal fatigue is that copper builds up in the body. It amplifies the emotions, and can trigger panic attacks, mood swings, schizophrenia and bipolar disorder. Emotional instability can be brought on through the presence of toxic metals such as cadmium, lead and mercury.

~ Symptoms of Adrenal Fatigue ~

[] weight gain (especially around the abdomen)
[] exhaustion
[] caffeine dependence
[] irregular menstrual cycles, e.g., bleeding for three days, not bleeding on the fourth day, then bleeding for days five and six
[] muscle/joint pain
[] craving salt
[] headaches
[] low libido
[] weakness
[] lethargy
[] dizziness
[] memory problems
[] food cravings, especially salt
[] allergies
[] blood sugar disorders
[] often complain of being cold
[] insomnia ~ fall asleep, then wake up several hours later and can't go back to sleep
[] even a small amount of stress makes you feel anxious and angry
[] recurring infections
[] respiratory problems such as asthma and allergies
[] slow to recover from sickness
[] low blood pressure

[] feeling faint when standing from a sitting position
[] low moods
[] minimal interest in life
[] you lack interest in things that used to make you feel happy
[] stimulants, such as coffee, needed to provide a boost of energy
[] hot flashes, night sweats, or PMT
[] sighing a lot
[] brown patches on the face and neck

Continued elevated cortisol levels are linked with: breast cancer, bone loss, heart disease, poor sleep quality, depression, Alzheimer's, infertility, blood sugar problems, decreased DHEA, fat accumulation, compromised immune function, inflammatory conditions and osteoporosis.

~ The Adrenal Glands ~

The outer portion of the glands ~ the adrenal cortex ~ produces cortisone. It helps with the metabolism of carbohydrates and in the regulation of blood sugar. It secretes a sex hormone. If it's underactive, it's known as *Addison's disease*.

If it's overactive, it's known as *Cushing's syndrome*.

The inner portion is called the adrenal medulla, and produces epinephrine (or adrenalin) and norepinephrine. Adrenalin is produced when the body is in a high stress condition.

The main factors which contribute to impaired adrenal function include: chronic stress, cortisone therapy for nonendocrine diseases (such as arthritis and asthma), pituitary diseases, tuberculosis, poor nutritional habits, smoking, alcohol, drugs, stress, depression, caffeine, and high-stress foods (such as fatty, fried and/or processed foods; sugar and red meat).

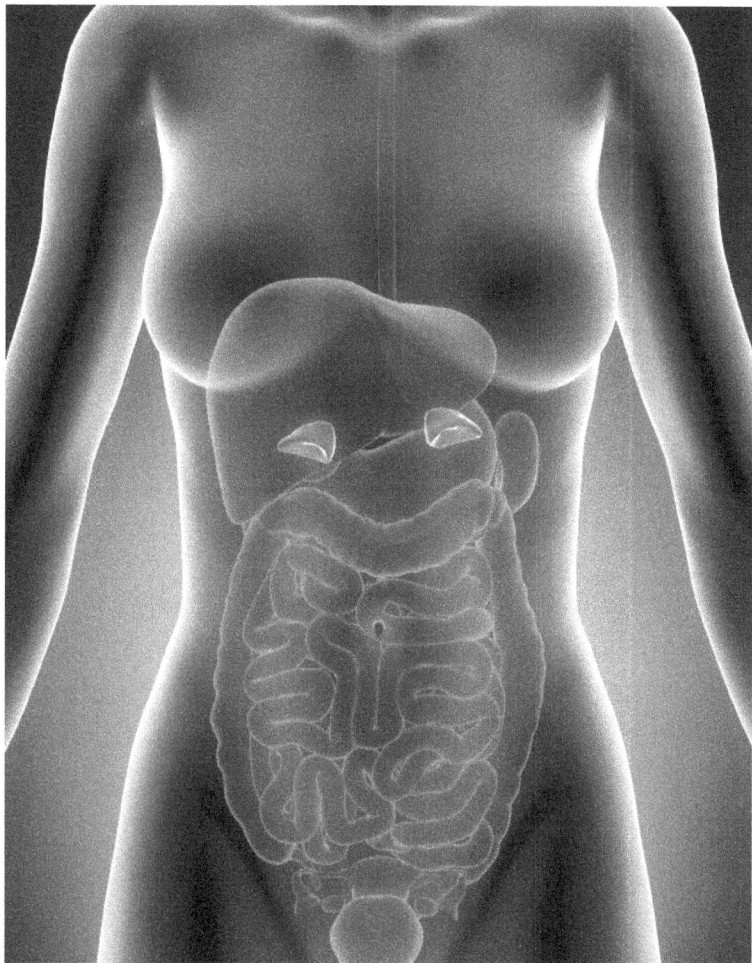

The adrenal glands sit on top of the kidneys.

~ Cortisol ~

One of the main hormones that the adrenals produce is cortisol. (The adrenals also produce other hormones such as DHEA, androstenedione, testosterone, oestrogen and progesterone).

Cortisol is what gets us out of bed in the morning, and able to function throughout the day. It is when we have too much of this pumping through our body, due to things like children fighting, road rage, financial stress, relationship worries and so on, that the problems start.

If we live in a constant state of high cortisol, we start to feel the effects.

The adrenals sit right above our kidneys, and act with all the other glands, especially the thyroid. They work together to maintain balance within the body. Unfortunately, ongoing stress will block many other processes from happening in the body.

When we go into "fight or flight", the body will go into natural preservation mode:
* storing fat
* shutting down any other non life-threatening processes in order to survive.

One of the effects is low thyroid function. This equals:

[] you gain loads of weight
[] have absolutely NO energy
[] hair loss
[] zero sex drive
[] infertility
[] feel cold all the time
[] increased oestrogen levels, which can lead to fibroids, cysts, cancers, irregular periods, PMT, out of control emotions
[] It's important to heal adrenal fatigue before menopause, as the adrenals take over at that time when the ovaries decrease production. If the adrenals are exhausted, the worst symptoms of menopause will occur.

~ Adrenal Fatigue Myths ~

[] You just need a holiday

Recovering from adrenal fatigue can take months or years, and won't be cured with two weeks on a Hawaiian beach! The relaxation WILL be good for you, but a brief change in your lifestyle will not fix everything up overnight.

[] It's an executive's illness

This is absolutely not true. The person most likely to get adrenal fatigue is a mother who is holding down a job, and trying to 'do it all'. People from all walks of life, of both sexes, and all ages, are susceptible to adrenal fatigue. Unfortunately, even children are prone to it, due to all the toxins and pressures of modern living. Symptoms in children include: chronic ear infections, cot death, ADHD, anti-social behaviour, brain dysfunction and failure to thrive.

[] It's all in the mind

No, it's all in the body. Adrenal fatigue is caused by the breaking down of the body's energy systems. As a result, essential minerals are lost, to be replaced by toxic metals. Fatigue is the biochemical reaction to ongoing stress, and affects behaviour and emotions. We can only heal when we recognise new ways of dealing with the psychological problems which triggered it.

[] You won't be able to hold down a job

Many people with adrenal fatigue still work full-time, reliant on stimulants such as coffee, spicy food, vigorous exercise and sugar.

[] Exercise will banish adrenal fatigue

Yes, some exercise is very helpful, but vigorous exercise is just another stimulant. The adrenal glands can't heal if they're exhausted through exercise.

[] You just need a good night's sleep

One of the main symptoms of adrenal fatigue is feeling worn out after a night of sleep. The body just doesn't seem to recharge itself. You often wake up more exhausted than when you went to bed!

It can be several years after a trauma before we notice adrenal fatigue. Adrenal exhaustion provides the foundation for degenerative disease. ALL illnesses begin with exhaustion, that is why it's imperative to find a natural, gentle, long-term healing route.

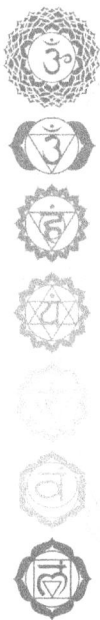

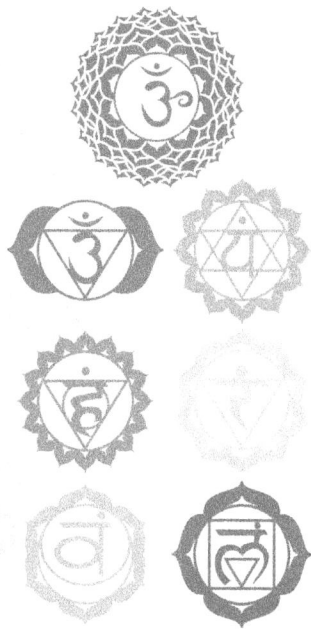

Meditation and yoga are beneficial for finding equilibrium.

~ My Healing Plan ~

This is what I wrote for myself when I began my healing journey to recovery. I'll go into more detail at the end of the list.

When I established everything that my body was going to need for healing, I wrote up a list and put it by my laptop ~ it was the very place it needed to be.

*Put my healing BEFORE my work
*Do something FUN each day
*Reclaim space for solitude and quiet
*Drink celery juice
*Drink 8 glasses of water every day
*Drink valerian, nettle and starflower tea
*Bee pollen
*Have protein smoothies
*Green superfood smoothies
*Vitamin C, B complex, E, trace minerals
*Astragalus
*Siberian ginseng
*Go to bed by 9pm most nights
*NO caffeine, chocolate or tannin
*Listen to more music
*Set firm boundaries
*Remove any source of stress
*Deep breathing & meditation

*Sit in the garden every day, no matter the weather
*Daily walks
*Rebounding
*Yoga and Pilates
*Coconut oil

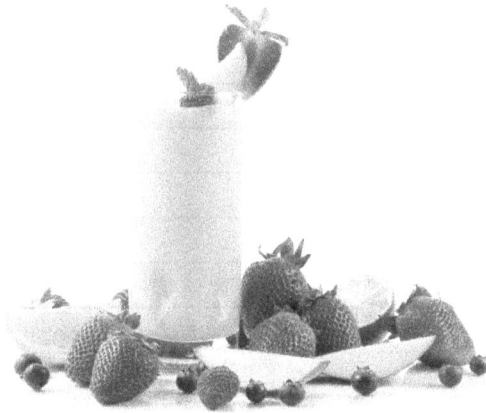

Write a list of how you intend to make healing adrenal fatigue your priority.

_____

_____

_____

_____

_____

_____

_____

_____

_____

_____

_____

_____

_____

_____

_____

_____

_____

_____

_____

_____

_____

_____

_____

_____

_____

_____

Put my healing BEFORE my work

Well, this one was easier said than done! I'm self-employed, and so the success of our business rests on my husband and I. Working seven days a week is normal for us. Over time I've learnt to 'let go' of the compulsion to work, and always ensure that I spend as much time as I can in the garden immersed in Nature. And if I have to work, where possible, I bring my editing or proofreading outside with me into the sunshine where I can be bathed in birdsong with my bare feet on the grass.

I no longer allow myself to feel obligated to answer emails on the day they arrive. I work to my own schedule.

Do something FUN each day

My teenage daughter starts each day with the question: "What are we doing that's fun today?" Everyone has a different idea of fun. My pleasures are simple: a long, hot bath; reading a book; going for a walk in country lanes; watching a rom-com.

In high school I used to read Mills & Boon romance novels every day ~ anything to alleviate

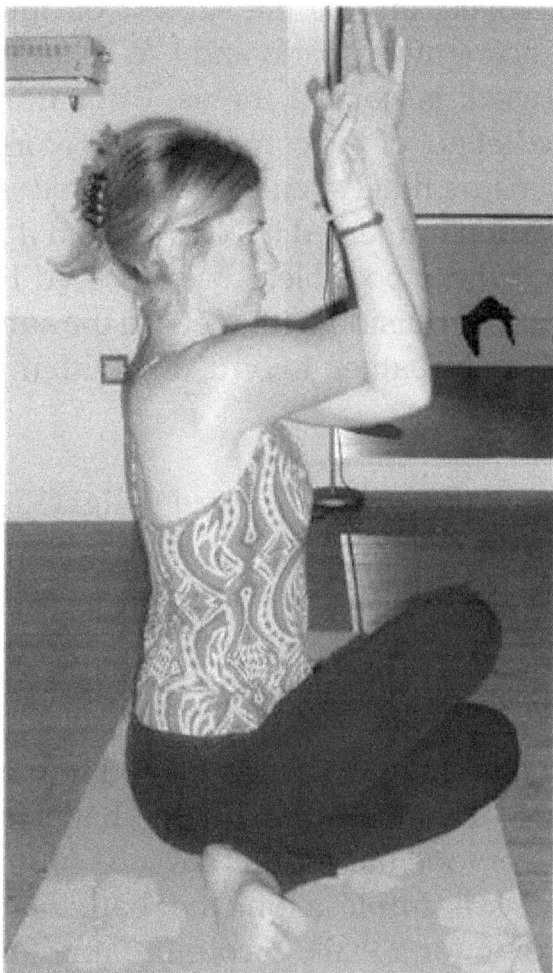

My friend, Jamie, doing yoga.

Write a list of fun things you love to do which you can incorporate in your day-to-day life.

_____
_____
_____
_____
_____
_____
_____
_____
_____
_____
_____
_____
_____
_____
_____
_____
_____
_____
_____
_____
_____
_____
_____
_____
_____
_____

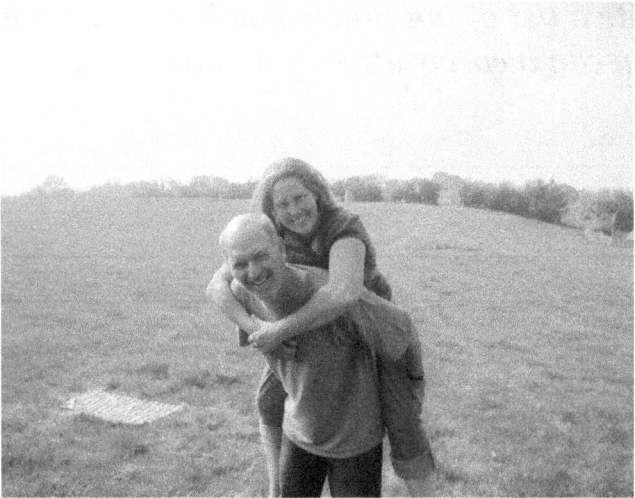

the boredom of maths and science! My daughters bought me a whole stack of these books during the month I was in bed ~ my older daughter was appalled that I read such basic literature... but, it was just what I needed. I'm used to reading heavy texts, and rarely read fiction of any description. These lightweight books were perfect.

Discover what your pleasures are, and be sure to include them each day. Just make sure they're not adrenal stressors! No climbing Mt. Everest, okay?

My husband Paul had always wanted to draw cartoons, and when he too developed adrenal fatigue he decided to take up this hobby. He started picking up the guitar more regularly, too.

Reclaim space for solitude and quiet

Because I work from home with my husband, and we home-educate our teenage daughters, solitude is something I have to create, each and every day. If we have adrenal fatigue, it's necessary to find this space in our healing so that we can look within: to find why we create certain behavioural patterns. It's very easy to surround ourselves with people and activities so that we never have to wander into the inner terrain and face our demons.

Drink celery juice

Celery juice is Nature's answer to ensuring we get the best form of sodium. Buy fresh, organic celery (or grow your own!), and juice a head of celery each day. According to Dr. Norman Walker, celery juice is the best way to heal the adrenals. *Read Fresh Vegetable and Fruit Juices, by Dr. Norman Walker.*

What can I do to create quiet, peace and solitude into each day?

_____

_____

_____

_____

_____

_____

_____

_____

_____

_____

_____

_____

_____

_____

_____

_____

_____

_____

_____

_____

_____

_____

_____

Drink 8 glasses of water every day

Recovering from just about every ailment and illness known to man is served well by the daily consumption of non-chemicalised water. Our body is made of approximately 80 to 90% water, but this percentage decreases the older we get. We literally shrivel up like prunes. But we don't have to! Nurture your insides by having water throughout the day. Read *Your Body's Many Cries for Water, by F. Batmanghelidj, M.D. www.watercure.com*

Drink valerian, nettle and starflower teas

Valerian tea is a relaxant, and calms the nervous system.

Nettle is rich in iron.

Starflower supports the adrenals. Make friends with these herbal teas, and ditch the coffee!

Starflower, is also known as borage, and grows so eas-

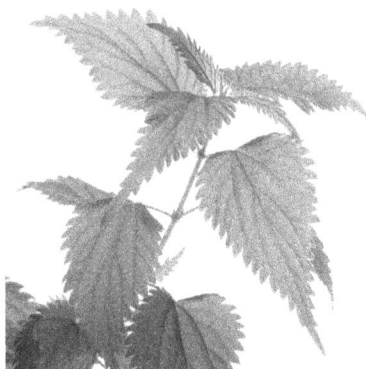

ily. Plant a few seeds in your garden and it will come up every year. You can make tea using fresh leaves, or dry them and store them for use throughout the Winter and Spring. Alternatively, buy your tea leaves here:
www.starflowerpress.com

Have protein smoothies

"Vegetarians don't recover from adrenal fatigue." I wasn't sure whether to laugh or cry when I read this advice in a mainstream book on adrenal fatigue cures. In truth, it was this absurd statement that prompted me to write this booklet. Why? Because there are so many myths about protein, and that vegetarians are lacking in amino acids.

Protein is a term which covers 22 organic compounds known as *amino acids*. Our body is able to synthesise many of these acids. The remaining eight, known as *essential amino acids*, must come from our diet.

Protein is found throughout the body in the form of hair, nails, bones, red blood cells and muscle tissue. The body requires it to build and repair tissue, carry nutrients, and for hormonal function. Protein comes from the Greek word:

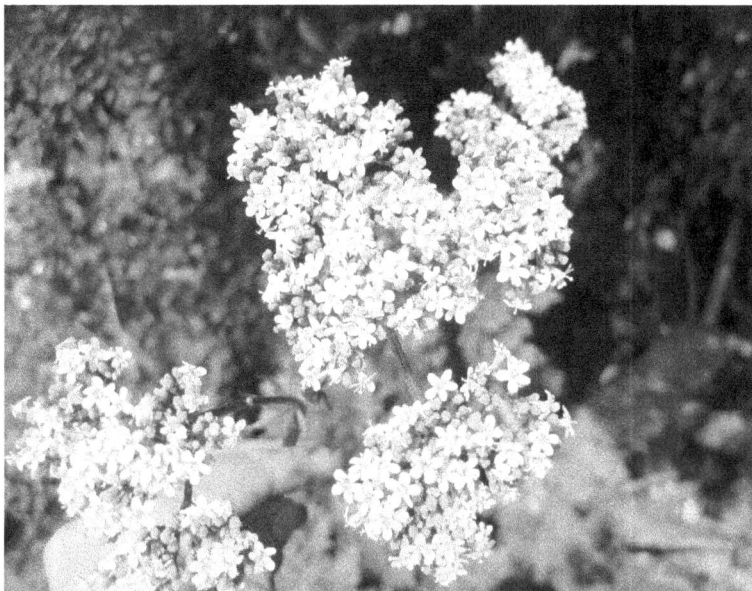

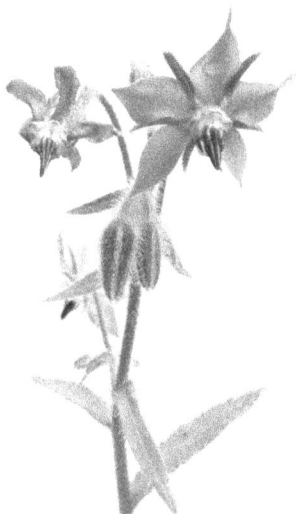

The root of the valerian (top) is used to make tea. Starflower (below) is made into tea from dried leaves and flowers. It's excellent for the adrenals.

What liquids do I regularly consume?
Do they support my adrenals?
How can I improve my liquid diet?

_____

_____

_____

_____

_____

_____

_____

_____

_____

_____

_____

_____

_____

_____

_____

_____

_____

_____

_____

_____

_____

_____

_____

_____

_____

_____

proteios, which means: of first quality. One third of our body's dry weight comes in the form of muscles; one fifth in bone and cartilage; and one tenth in skin. The rest is made up of tissue, body fluids and blood.

As a vegetarian child growing up in beef cattle country, in Queensland, Australia, I heard the phrase 'you'll die if you don't eat meat' more often than I care to remember. That I didn't die from protein deficiency must surely be a miracle. Right? Wrong.

In the Western world, we've been brainwashed into believing that we're at risk of not getting enough protein if we don't eat meat. Vegetarians are always given the advice that plant-based proteins are inadequate, and therefore they must 'combine' proteins. Let's look at these two myths closely: there's no *factual* basis for the belief that a high-protein diet is necessary for good health. It's an ungrounded fear conveniently propounded by the meat and dairy industries. It's been repeated so often that just about everyone believes it to be true.

The meat industry led us to believe that we need about 120 grams of protein a day. This information came out of Germany at the start of the last century. Nowadays, we know that a human needs more like 20 to 35 grams a day. In fact, only about 2.5% of our daily calorie intake should come from proteins.

Breast milk has about 5% of its calories coming from protein.

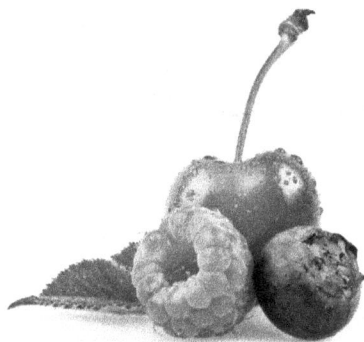

In the 1980s, the idea of food combining to obtain the right protein was made popular. It was probably from this that fear-mongering for vegetarians really set in, because people were concerned that they weren't getting 'complete' proteins.

What we now know is that humans store protein, so combining is unnecessary. As with any

What do I believe about protein?
What protein do I include in my diet?

_____

_____

_____

_____

_____

_____

_____

_____

_____

_____

_____

_____

_____

_____

_____

_____

_____

_____

_____

_____

_____

_____

_____

_____

_____

diet, variety is the key, and this is no different for a vegetarian diet. Unless such a diet is laden with junk foods and sugar, there's absolutely no reason for it to be deficient in protein. And the more living (raw) foods which are included, the more protein is available, as about half of the assimilable protein is destroyed during cooking.

Over-consumption of animal protein, which is common in Western society, results in heart disease, cancer, kidney damage, arthritis, pyorrhea, schizophrenia and atherosclerosis, as well as premature aging.

Overconsumption of meat leads to cell, organ and tissue degeneration, and amyloid deposits. This all creates an acidic system.

There's overwhelming evidence that decreasing the amount of protein in a diet (that is, removing meat) can prevent osteoporosis. Research into protein intake shows that consuming 75g a day or more draws calcium from the bones.

Protein absorption is inhibited by fizzy liquids, antacids and baking soda.

Sources of ethical protein:
all leafy greens (these are the foundation of life on our planet)
most fruits
soybeans
tofu
sunflower seeds
pumpkin seeds
sesame seeds
almonds
buckwheat
Mila (a mix of chia seeds)
quinoa
breast milk
amaranth
millet
pollen, if sourced from a shamanic beekeeper, is an excellent source of protein, as well as all the other nutrients a human needs. See www.kiki-health.co.uk

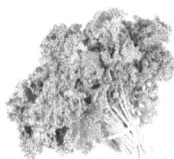

Green superfood smoothies

Green. Think green. The more green you can include in your diet, the better. Think of things like kelp, spirulina, chlorella, sea vegetables, E3 live (blue-green algae). Because of the likelihood of your thyroid being impaired by adrenal fatigue, I recommend having kelp every day. I open up the capsules and put the powder into my smoothies.

Vitamin C, B complex, E, trace minerals

Many commercial vitamin C tablets have so many horrific ingredients that I'm shocked they're allowed to be sold. I recommend Truly Natural vitamin C; and Biocare's liquid vitamin B. Trace minerals, I obtain from Himalayan Pink Salt. (*www.detoxyourworld.com*)

Astragalus

This is one of the most important remedies for nourishing the adrenals. Buy it in tincture form. The two brands I've used are Postlethwaites organic, and Swiss Herbal Remedies. More about astragalus on page 57.
www.postlethwaites.co.uk

Siberian ginseng

Siberian ginseng is deeply nourishing to anyone who's healing from an illness. It's an adaptogen, which means it works with the body, rather than on a specific part of it. Floradix provides this in a liquid tonic. More about Siberian ginseng on page 58.

What can I do to create a 'nest' for night-time,
so that I look forward to going to sleep?
Is my bedroom inviting and calming, and free
from stressors, such as: an alarm clock, work,
digital clock radio with garish LCD,
mobile phone, and so on?

_____

_____

_____

_____

_____

_____

_____

_____

_____

_____

_____

_____

_____

_____

_____

_____

_____

_____

_____

_____

_____

Go to bed by 9pm most nights

I found this so hard to achieve, because I look forward to the evenings as a quiet time to get work done or write books. But if you've got adrenal fatigue and you want to get better, you need to develop new habits, and going to bed early is one of them.

No caffeine, chocolate or tannin

And even harder than going to bed early was giving up coffee! It's not even that I had that much of it...a cup a day is my maximum, and two at most, but only if before lunchtime. Caffeine keeps me awake all night, so I know that to live with this sensitivity I have to keep my consumption down. However, even with one cup, I still felt I needed it to get through the day. I tried being clever and switching to hot chocolate ~ the lovely organic pure cacao, but that was just as bad. Even Earl Grey tea keeps me awake all night. The bottom line is that any of these stimulants are not conducive to healing the adrenals and they have to go if you're serious about recovery. Try dandelion coffee, Barley cup and herbal or fruit teas. Best of all, drink plenty of pure water.

Listen to more music

Music is a wonderful tool to aid relaxation, assuming it's pleasant, like baroque, and not Lady Gaga. Use this time to explore new musical genres, and find what relaxes you.

I've also begun learning to play the cello, and find this very relaxing.

Set firm boundaries

Many of us have grown up to be people pleasers. The most helpful advice I can ever give is this: *When you say "no" to others, you're saying "yes" to yourself.* To heal adrenal fatigue, you'll need to learn the art of saying "Yes" to YOU. You deserve it, and crucially, you need to come first. Be wary of people who drain what little energy you have.

Remove any source of stress

Be honest with yourself about *all* stressors, and one by one minimise or eliminate them. You have an illness, and need healing time.

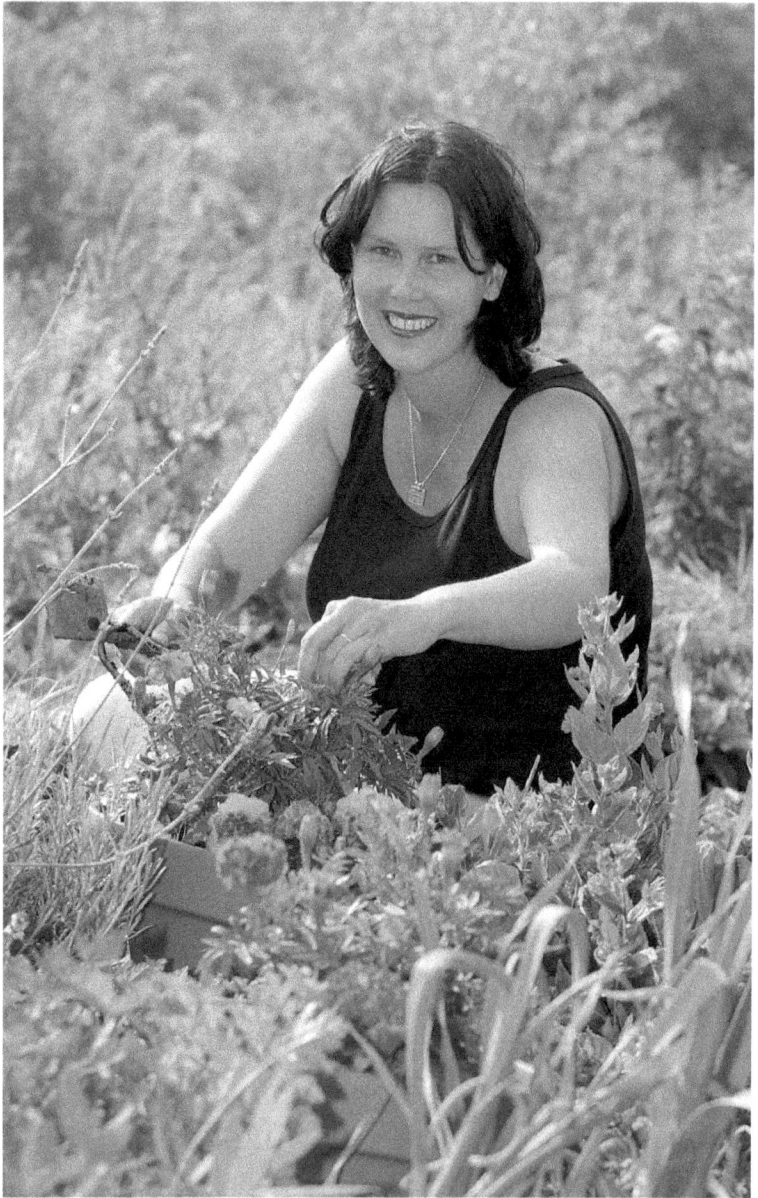

Whether you're a gardener or not, make time each day to enjoy being amongst the flowers, birdsong, sunshine and fresh air.

Deep breathing & meditation

We breathe 20,000 times a day, but rarely give it any thought. Learning to breathe deeply, especially in fresh air, will bring calmness to your body.

There are many ways to meditate. Learn the art of stillness and quiet contemplation.

Sit in the garden every day

Regardless of the time of year, sit in your garden (or nearby park) and just be 'one' with Nature. Allow yourself to breathe deeply, and let go of all worrying thoughts. If you must think, find something pleasant to occupy your mind. What we think about most of the time becomes our life.

Daily walks

I've always enjoyed walking, and make sure I walk three miles a day.

Rebounding

Rebounding on a mini-trampoline is a fantastic exercise as it stimulates the lymphatic sys-

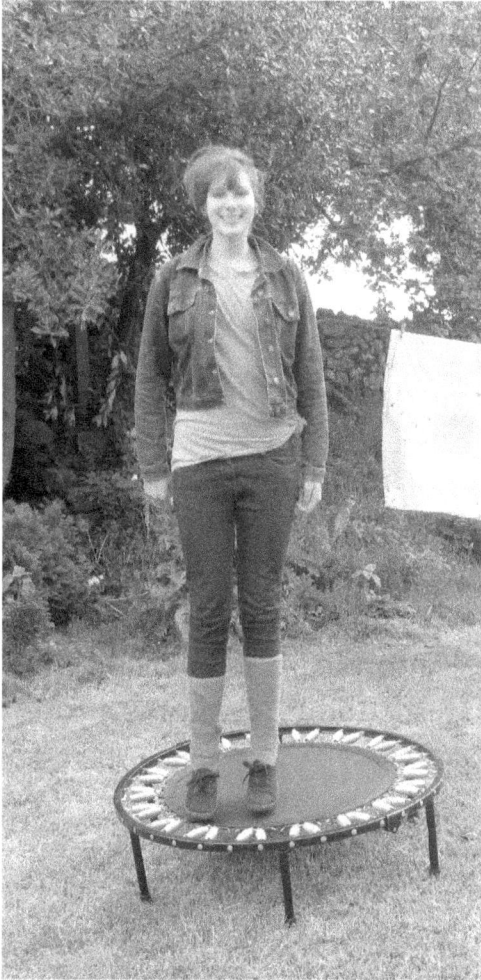

My daughter, Bethany, enjoying a bounce on the rebounder. It stimulates the lymphatic system, which allows detoxing. It's a gentle exercise for those with adrenal fatigue.

tem, which is essential for detoxing. It's easy to do, and very gentle. It exercises every muscle in the body. Ten minutes a day is equivalent to 20 minutes jogging, without the sweat! I can't recommend it highly enough. Rebounding is a beautiful way to start the day.

Yoga and Pilates

A gentle yoga, such as Yin Yoga, is incredibly relaxing, and will allow the nervous system to function optimally.

Pilates is another gentle way to exercise the entire body. If you've put on abdominal weight, a regular programme will help you to support your core muscles. Join a class, or find a good teacher and have a one-on-one session to have a programme devised for your specific needs.

Coconut oil

Coconut oil is a wonderful cure for many ailments which afflict the body, adrenal fatigue and low thyroid being two of them. Simply change your cooking oil to coconut, or eat it straight off the teaspoon. In my experience, the only brand I like is Biona's organic coconut oil. It's raw and unbleached.

Homeopathy

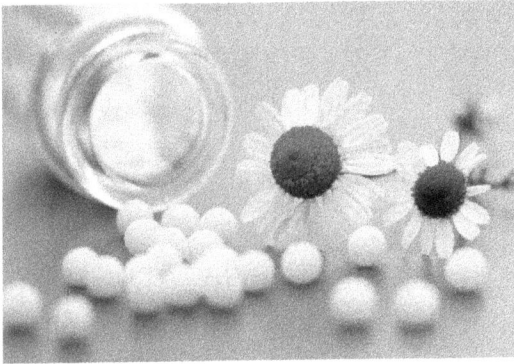

I took three homeopathic remedies for healing from adrenal exhaustion. I identified a time in my life, some years before, when most of the symptoms, apart from exhaustion, started. I'd been involved in a court case to defend the right-of-way deed to my property. The extreme stress, eventual bankruptcy, and the end decision to sell the land caused a lot of grief. This was the trigger to my exhaustion four years later. Some people have a shock, and the adrenals immediately collapse.

Oak 6x

This is for exhaustion, but having to keep going. It's powerfully grounding and energising. Think of the oak tree's strength.

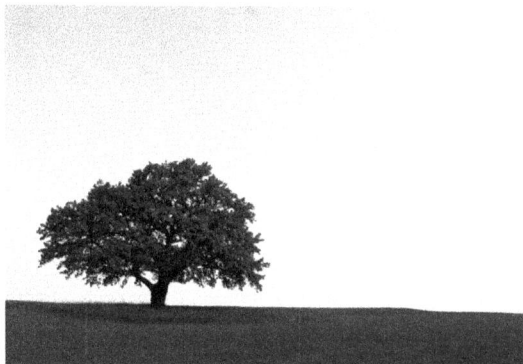

Sycamore Seed 12c

Specific for the adrenal glands, as it supports glands in pairs. You can see the *'doctrine of signatures'*** (see page 60) when you look at the seeds.

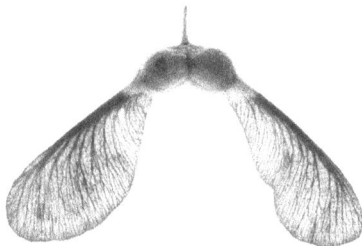

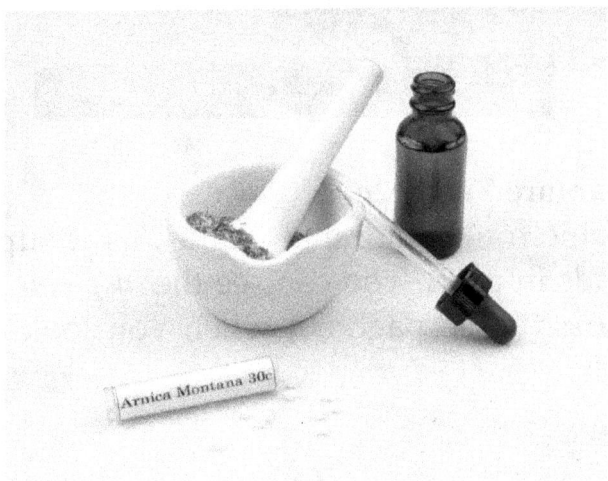

Arnica Montana 30c

Phos-ac 30c

This is for exhaustion with the aetiology of grief.

Many homeopathic remedies are based on lactose (the sugar in cows' milk). I had mine made free of lactose.

I also found that meditating on the sycamore seeds was a powerful part of my visualisations. I often pick up these 'angel wings' when out on my daily walks.

Ancient Hawaiian Healing

Ho'oponopono is the ancient Hawaiian healing technique based on forgiveness. It is based on four lines:

I love you
I'm sorry
Please forgive me (for whatever it is inside me that's causing me to experience adrenal fatigue)
Thank you.

Please forgive me means forgiving yourself for the false thoughts.
Thank you acknowledges that healing has begun. You can use this for anything in your life. Say it as often as you like throughout the day.
http://www.whatishooponopono.com/ Hooponopono_Dr_Ihaleakala_Hew_Len.htm

Healing modalities:

There are various healing modalities you can introduce. The two which have helped me are reflexology (specific to adrenals and thyroid), and chiropractic (which releases tension to the nervous system, thereby allowing the body to heal).

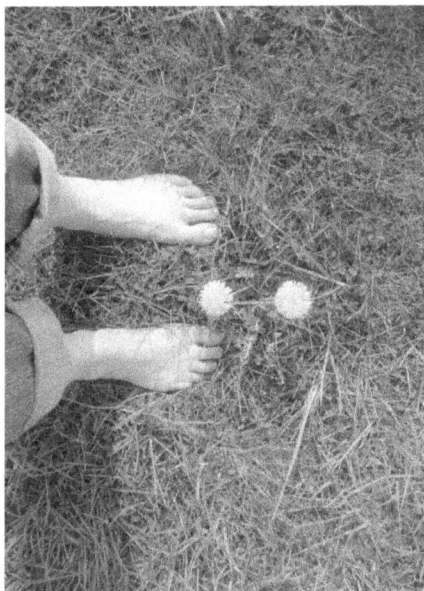

Grounding

Where possible, try and walk barefoot on the earth (grass, dirt, sand) for at least half an hour a day as this is incredibly healing to the human body. We spend our lives with our feet 'blind-folded', and unable to read the natural world around us. *See www.earthing.com*

You might like to try:
cranio-sacral therapy
homeopathy
herbal healing
acupuncture

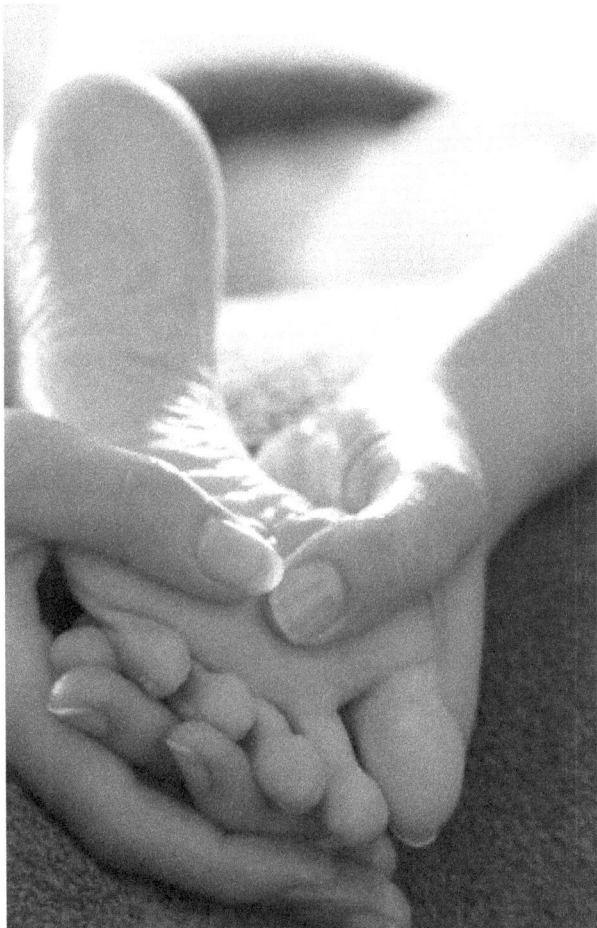

Reflexology

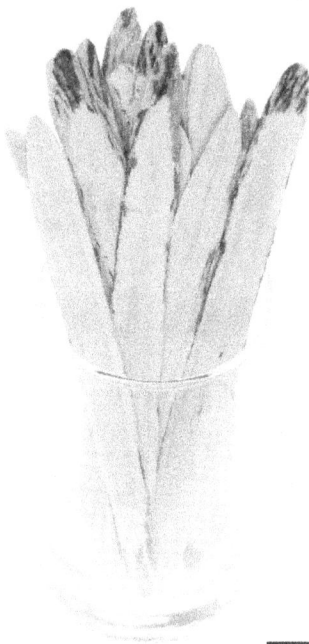

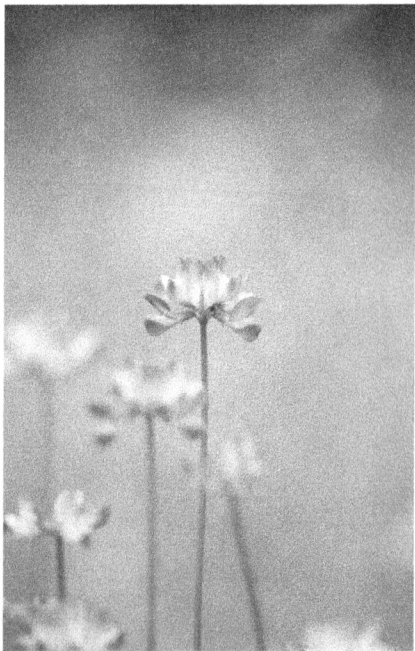

Above: astragalus root.
Below: astragalus in flower.

~ Astragalus ~

Astragalus is one of the main herbs to use in healing the adrenals. Use it in combination with Siberian ginseng. Astragalus is antibacterial, and generates warming energy. It bolsters the white blood cell count, and strengthens the body's resistance.

Scientists have isolated a number of active ingredients contained in astragalus, including bioflavanoids, choline, and a polysaccharide called astragalan B.

Astragalus is well known for the way it strengthens and supports the immune system.

~ Siberian Ginseng Root ~
(Eleutherococcus senticosus)

Siberian ginseng isn't strictly a ginseng, or, ironically, from Siberia. It's well known for supporting and helping to rejuventate the adrenals. It increases one's resistance to stress. Siberian ginseng normalises metabolism, and regulates neurotransmitters. It increases energy levels, endurance, stamina, and counteracts mental fatigue. It is used to calm anxiousness, diminish lethargy, act as an antidepressant, help with sleeping, and promotes a sense of well-being. Its ability to increase vitality helps to counter the effects of the adrenal stress hormones while normalising blood sugar levels, increasing resistance to pollutants in the environment, and stimulating antibodies. Vitamins B and C are absorbed more effectively when Siberian ginseng is consumed.

~ Food Choices ~

Natural: Avoid refined, processed, high-stress foods, and preservatives, artificial colours and flavours.

Locally-grown: The most healthy way to eat is to have as much locally-grown, in-season produce as you can.

Wild-crafted
Where possible, choose foods which have been grown in the wild.

Organic
If you're unable to source wild foods, then choose organic or those grown without chemicals.

Peaceful dining
Ensure your meals are eaten in a calm and peaceful environment so you don't create even more stress while you're eating. If you eat under stress, your body will not be able to absorb nutrients.

Water
Drink plenty of fresh, pure, clean water every day.

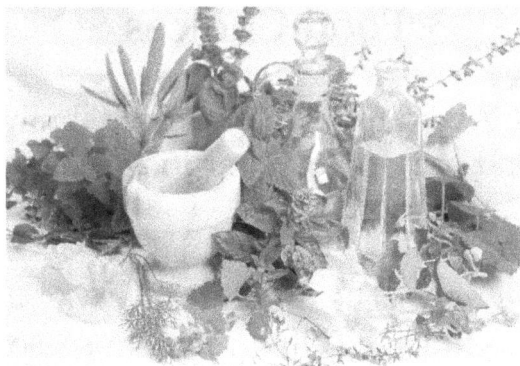

Healing

You can't hurry the healing of the adrenal glands. Allow at least two years to get any sense of 'normality' back. It involves commitment and dedication to your well-being, and will require a complete overhaul of diet, lifestyle and how you deal with emotional toxins.

I wish you an insightful, peaceful and healing journey.

** The *Doctrine of Signatures* is a very old notion and was mentioned in the writings of the Swiss physician, Paracelsus von Hohenheim (1493-1541). It proposes the idea that God gave everything in Nature its unique healing powers, and left a clue for us to discover in the appearance of each plant or substance.

~ My Adrenal Symptoms ~

_____

_____

_____

_____

_____

_____

_____

_____

_____

_____

_____

_____

_____

_____

_____

_____

_____

_____

_____

_____

_____

_____

_____

_____

_____

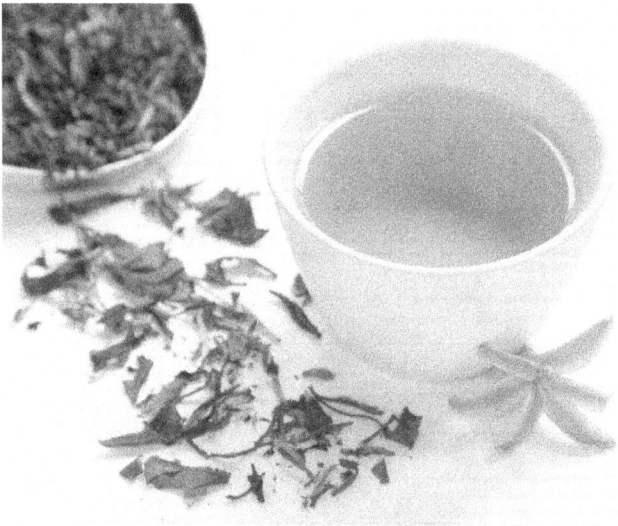

~ My Healing Notes ~

_____
_____
_____
_____
_____
_____
_____
_____
_____
_____
_____
_____
_____
_____
_____
_____
_____
_____
_____
_____
_____
_____
_____
_____
_____
_____
_____
_____

~ My Healing Notes ~

_____

_____

_____

_____

_____

_____

_____

_____

_____

_____

_____

_____

_____

_____

_____

_____

_____

_____

_____

_____

_____

_____

_____

_____

_____

_____

_____

_____

_____

~ My Healing Notes ~

_____
_____
_____
_____
_____
_____
_____
_____
_____
_____
_____
_____
_____
_____
_____
_____
_____
_____
_____
_____
_____
_____
_____
_____
_____
_____
_____
_____
_____

~ Resources ~

Vitamins and minerals

Your local health shop should be able to provide you with the following, otherwise try: www.detoxyourworld.com

[] Biocare liquid vitamin B

[] Viridian kelp

[] Viridian vitamin D

[] Biona's organic raw coconut oil

[] Truly Natural Acerola Cherry
(Health Force Nutritionals)

[] Olive leaf extract
www.OliveLeafComplex.com

[] Mila (whole raw chia seeds)
Lifemax.net

[] Bee pollen (avoid capsules, and source freshly frozen pollen) See Kiki Limited.

[] Himalayan pink salt www.detoxyourworld.com

~ Reading ~

Coconut Cures, *by Dr. Bruce Fife.*

Olive Leaf Extract, *by Jack Ritchason, ND*

Fresh Vegetable and Fruit Juices: what's missing in your body?, *by Dr. Norman Walker*

http://www.whatishooponopono.com/Hooponopono_Dr_Ihaleakala_Hew_Len.htm

Earthing: The Most Important Health Discovery Ever?, *by Clinton Ober, Stephen Sinatra and Martin Zucker*

~ About the Publisher ~

Starflower Press is dedicated to publishing material which lifts the heart, and helps to raise human consciousness to a new level of awareness.

It draws its name and inspiration from the olden-day herb, Borage (Borago Officinalis), commonly known as Starflower, which is still found in many places, though it's often thought of as a wild flower, rather than a herb.

Starflower is recognisable by its beautiful star-like flowers, which are formed by five petals of intense blue (sometimes they're pink). The unusual blue colour was used in Renaissance paintings. The Biblical meaning of this blue is heavenly grace.

Borage, from the Celtic *borrach*, means courage. Throughout history, Starflower has been associated with courage. It's used as a food, tea, tincture and flower essence to bring joy to the heart, and gladden the mind.

Visit www.starflowerpress.com

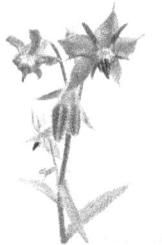

www.ingramcontent.com/pod-product-compliance
Lightning Source LLC
Chambersburg PA
CBHW060632280326
41933CB00012B/2016